KIDNEY DIET COOKBOOK FOR SENIORS

Delicious and Nutritious Recipes for Health

Dr. Esther Emmanuel

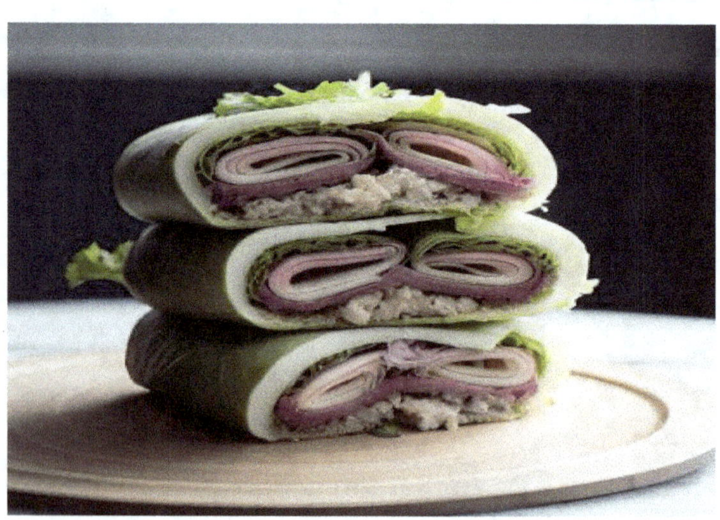

TABLE OF CONTENTS

INTRODUCTION

Mrs. Johnson had been struggling with kidney disease for years. She had tried every possible medication and treatment, but nothing seemed to work. The doctors had told her that she would have to live with this condition for the rest of her life. But then she discovered the power of diet therapy.

Mrs. Johnson had always been a foodie, but now she had to be more careful with what she ate. She consulted a dietitian and started following a strict diet plan that was designed specifically for her condition. She had to cut down on her favorite foods, such as red meat, dairy products, and processed foods. Instead, she had to consume more fruits, vegetables, whole grains, and lean proteins.

At first, it was difficult for Mrs. Johnson to adjust to this new diet. She missed her old foods and felt frustrated. But she knew that she had to stick to it if she wanted to get better. Slowly but surely, she started feeling the difference. Her energy levels increased, and her overall health improved.

After a few months, Mrs. Johnson went back to her doctor for a routine check-up. To her surprise, her doctor was amazed by the progress she had made. Her kidney function had improved significantly, and her blood pressure had stabilized. Her doctor couldn't believe it and asked her what she had been doing differently.

Mrs. Johnson told her doctor about her new diet plan and how it had transformed her health. Her doctor was impressed and encouraged her to keep it up. Mrs. Johnson felt ecstatic. She couldn't believe that something as simple as changing her diet could have such a profound impact on her health.

Over time, Mrs. Johnson became an advocate for diet therapy. She shared her story with anyone who would listen, encouraging them to adopt healthy eating habits. She even started a blog where she shared her favorite recipes and tips for maintaining a healthy diet.

Mrs. Johnson's journey wasn't easy, but it was worth it. She learned that taking care of her body was the most important thing she could do for herself. She no longer felt like a victim of her disease but rather like a survivor who had taken control of her health.

In the end, Mrs. Johnson's story inspired many others to take charge of their health. She had shown them that it was possible to heal through diet therapy and that they didn't have to rely solely on medications to feel better.

Mrs. Johnson's journey had not only transformed her life, but it had also touched the lives of countless others.

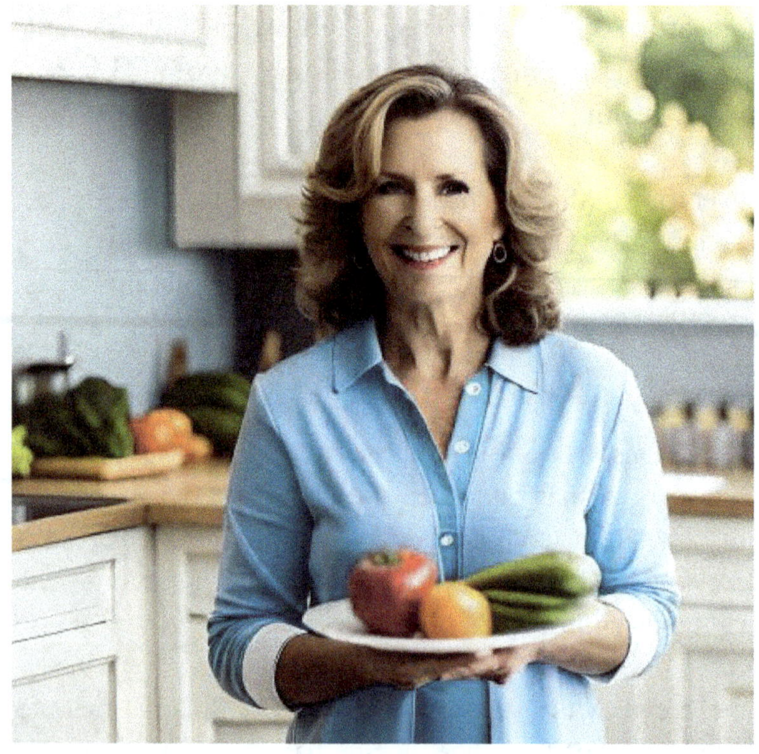

CHAPTER 1

KIDNEY-FRIENDLY FOODS FOR SENIORS

A renal-friendly diet is crucial to the management of kidney disease in older people. A kidney-friendly diet aims to lessen the burden on the kidneys, prevent the accumulation of waste, and keep the body's fluid and electrolyte levels in a healthy range. Several senior-friendly diets for the kidneys include:

1. Fruits and veggies: Since they are low in phosphorus, potassium, and salt, fresh fruits and vegetables are fantastic options for elderly people with kidney disease. Fruits and vegetables including apples, blueberries, strawberries, cucumbers, green beans, and carrots are examples of those that are good for the kidneys.

2. Dairy items with low fat: Dairy products with low fat, like milk, yogurt, and cheese, are a healthy source of calcium and protein, but older adults with kidney disease should take them in moderation. Avoid high-phosphorus dairy items like cheese spreads and flavored yogurts and opt for low- or non-fat alternatives.

3. Lean protein: Protein is essential for seniors, however choosing lean types of protein will help to lessen the strain on the kidneys. Chicken, fish, eggs, and tofu are a few examples of protein foods that are good for the kidneys.

4. Whole grains: Compared to refined grains, whole grains like quinoa, whole wheat bread, and brown rice are better sources of fiber and other nutrients and have lower potassium content.

5. Spices and herbs: Spices and herbs can flavor food without adding sodium. Basil, thyme, rosemary, and garlic are a few herbs and spices that are beneficial to the kidneys.

6. Water: Seniors with renal illness may need to restrict their fluid consumption because water is crucial for kidney function. Consult a healthcare professional to determine the best fluid intake depending on your unique needs.

Working with a qualified dietitian to create a custom kidney-friendly eating plan is crucial for elders with renal disease. A dietitian can offer assistance in identifying dietary requirements, monitoring nutritional levels, and advising on proper portion sizes.

Overview of a kidney-friendly diet

A kidney-friendly diet is a dietary strategy created to support people with kidney disease in keeping their health and halting the disease's progression. Reducing the stress on the kidneys, preventing the development of waste products in the body, and maintaining healthy levels of fluid and electrolytes are the basic objectives of a kidney-friendly diet.

Some broad suggestions for a kidney-friendly diet include the ones listed below:

1. Limit your sodium consumption since too much of it can cause high blood pressure, which can strain your kidneys even more. Seniors with renal illness should strive to consume no more than 2,300 mg of sodium per day.

2. Watch the amounts of potassium and phosphorus: Minerals like potassium and phosphorus can accumulate in the blood of people with renal disease. Bananas, oranges, avocados, dairy products, almonds, and other foods high in potassium and phosphorus may need to be avoided by seniors with kidney disease.

3. Pick the proper kinds of protein: Some protein sources can be harmful to the kidneys, although protein is necessary for maintaining muscle mass and general health. Lean forms of protein, like chicken, fish, eggs, and tofu, should be consumed by seniors with kidney disease.

4. Drink plenty of water: Seniors with renal illness may need to restrict their fluid consumption because water is crucial for kidney function. Consult a healthcare professional to determine the best fluid intake depending on your unique needs.

5. Limit your alcohol consumption because it can dehydrate you and raise your blood pressure, which is bad for your kidneys. Seniors with renal illness should consume alcohol in moderation or not at all.

Working with a qualified dietitian to create a custom kidney-friendly eating plan is crucial for elders with renal disease. A dietitian can offer assistance in identifying dietary requirements, monitoring nutritional levels, and advising on proper portion sizes.

The importance of a kidney-friendly diet for seniors

Seniors should eat kidney-friendly foods because developing kidney disease becomes more likely as people get older. Over 50% of persons over 65 have some form of renal disease, according to the National renal Foundation. Numerous health issues, such as fluid retention, electrolyte imbalances, and harm to the heart, blood vessels, and bones, can be brought on by kidney illness. A diet that is kidney-friendly for seniors can help them manage their kidney illness, stop future kidney damage, and enhance their general health.

Limiting some nutrients that can be damaging to the kidneys, such as salt, phosphorus, and potassium, while increasing the intake of nutrients that are good for kidney health, such as protein, fiber, and vitamins, is the norm for a renal-friendly diet for seniors.

For instance, sodium is frequently limited in a diet that is friendly to the kidneys because it can raise blood pressure and create fluid retention. Seniors with renal illness may also have negative effects from high phosphorus and potassium levels since these nutrients might exacerbate kidney dysfunction and accelerate bone resorption.

Protein, on the other hand, is crucial for preserving muscle mass and enhancing general health, but elderly people with renal disease may need to restrict their protein consumption to prevent their kidneys from being overworked. Fiber is crucial for kidney health because it helps lower blood sugar and cholesterol levels, both of which over time can harm the kidneys.

Seniors can manage various health concerns including high blood pressure, diabetes, and heart disease by eating a diet that is friendly to their kidneys. Seniors' general health and quality of life can be enhanced by eating a kidney-friendly diet, which can also help them maintain a healthy weight and control blood pressure.

In order to control their health and avoid complications, seniors who are receiving dialysis or who have had a kidney transplant may also need to adhere to a kidney-friendly diet. Seniors can work with a certified dietitian to create a customized kidney-friendly diet plan that takes into consideration their unique health requirements, preferences, and lifestyle.

Tips for following a kidney diet as a senior

Although adhering to a kidney diet can be difficult, it is crucial for elderly people with kidney disease to preserve their health and avoid problems. Here are some pointers for senior citizens on a kidney diet:

1. Working with a trained dietitian can help seniors create a customized kidney-friendly food plan that

takes into consideration their unique health requirements, preferences, and lifestyle. Additionally, a nutritionist can offer advice on meal planning, food selection, and portion sizes.

2. Read nutrition information on food labels: Seniors with kidney disease should be aware of the amount of nutrients in the food they consume. Seniors who read food labels can discover foods that are high in potassium, phosphorus, and sodium and make better food decisions.

3. Reduce sodium consumption: Seniors with renal disease should try to keep their daily sodium intake to under 2,300 mg. To do this, stay away from processed meals, season food with herbs and spices rather than salt, and pick low-sodium options when they are offered.

4. Seniors with kidney illness should pick proteins that are beneficial to their kidneys, such as lean meat, chicken, fish, and eggs. An eating plan that is good for the kidneys can also contain plant-based sources of protein such as beans, lentils, and tofu.

5. Limit phosphorus and potassium intake: Phosphorus and potassium, which are present in

high concentrations in dairy products, nuts, seeds, and some fruits and vegetables, should be avoided by seniors with kidney disease. A dietician can offer advice on which meals to limit or stay away from.

6. Stay hydrated: Seniors with renal illness should make an effort to consume enough fluids to stay hydrated, but they should also be careful not to consume too much fluid. A nutritionist can offer advice on how much liquids each person should consume.

7. Exercise frequently: Maintaining a healthy weight, lowering blood pressure, and enhancing general health are all possible for elderly people with kidney disease who routinely exercise. Before beginning an exercise regimen, seniors should speak with their doctor.

Although adhering to a kidney diet might be difficult, seniors with kidney disease can preserve their health and enhance their quality of life by working with a certified dietitian and making a few easy lifestyle changes.

Foods to limit or avoid for kidney health

Certain foods should be avoided or limited for those with renal disease to keep their kidneys healthy. These consist of:

1. High-sodium foods: Foods with a lot of sodium can raise blood pressure, which can strain the kidneys even more. Foods high in sodium, such as canned and processed foods, fast food, and salty snacks, should be avoided by seniors with kidney disease.

2. Foods high in potassium: People with kidney illness may have an accumulation of the mineral potassium in their blood. Foods high in potassium, such as bananas, oranges, avocados, tomatoes, potatoes, and dairy products, may need to be avoided by seniors with kidney disease.

3. High-phosphorus foods: People with kidney disease may experience a buildup of the mineral phosphorus in their blood. Foods high in phosphorus, such as dairy goods, nuts, legumes, and whole grains, should be avoided by seniors with kidney disease.

4. Foods high in protein: Protein helps maintain lean muscle mass and overall health, however some types of protein can be damaging to the kidneys. Red meat, processed meats, and high-protein dairy items should be avoided by senior citizens with kidney impairment.

5. Sugary meals and beverages: Consuming sugary foods and beverages can lead to weight increase, which can place additional stress on the kidneys. The consumption of sugary foods and beverages, such as soda, candy, and baked goods, should be restricted in seniors with kidney disease.

Working with a qualified dietitian to create a custom kidney-friendly eating plan is crucial for elders with renal disease. A dietitian can offer assistance in identifying dietary requirements, monitoring nutritional levels, and advising on proper portion sizes.

Foods to incorporate for kidney health

There are a number of foods that people with kidney disease can include in their diets to keep their kidneys healthy. These consist of:

1. Vegetables and fruits: Vegetables and fruits are a good source of fiber, vitamins, and minerals.

Seniors with renal illness should make an effort to eat a range of vibrant fruits and vegetables, such as bell peppers, squash, leafy greens, and berries.

2. Low-sodium foods: To lessen the strain on their kidneys, senior citizens with kidney disease should try to eat low-sodium foods. Lean meats, healthy grains, and fresh or frozen fruits and vegetables are all excellent low-sodium choices.

3. Low-phosphorus foods: To prevent the blood from becoming too phosphorus-rich, senior citizens with kidney disease should try to eat low-phosphorus foods. Foods low in phosphorus include fruits and vegetables, white bread, rice, and pasta.

4. Low-potassium foods: Although seniors with kidney illness may need to restrict their potassium intake, it's still crucial to include some low-potassium items in their diets. Apples, cabbage, green beans, and carrots are some examples of foods that are low in potassium.

5. Unsaturated fats, such those in nuts, avocados, and olive oil, can be integrated into the diet to support heart health and general wellbeing.

Working with a qualified dietitian to create a custom kidney-friendly eating plan is crucial for elders with renal disease. A dietitian can offer assistance in identifying dietary requirements, monitoring nutritional levels, and advising on proper portion sizes.

Tips for meal planning and portion control

Meal planning and portion control are crucial components of sustaining kidney health for seniors with kidney disease. Here are some pointers for organizing meals and managing portions:

1. Consult a certified dietitian: A registered dietitian can assist elderly people with kidney disease in creating a tailored meal plan that takes into consideration their unique dietary needs and constraints. Additionally, a nutritionist can offer advice on food preparation and quantity control.

2. Use measuring equipment: Seniors can control their portion sizes and make sure they are not overeating by using measuring spoons and cups. Protein portion measurements can also be made with the aid of a food scale.

3. Lean protein sources should be sought out by seniors with kidney disease, such as skinless

chicken, fish, and tofu. These protein sources are less likely to cause the blood to become clogged with waste materials.

4. Seniors with renal illness should watch their sodium consumption and try to reduce it. Intake of salt can be decreased by reading nutrition labels, selecting low-sodium choices, and preparing meals at home.

5. Include fruits and vegetables in your diet: Because they are high in vitamins and minerals and low in salt, fruits and vegetables are crucial components of a kidney-friendly diet. Seniors should make an effort to include a range of fruit and vegetable colors in their meals.

6. Choosing whole grains can help reduce your chance of developing heart disease because they are a rich source of fiber and minerals. Brown rice, quinoa, and whole wheat bread are examples of healthy grains that seniors with kidney disease should pick.

7. Reduce your intake of high-potassium foods: Seniors with renal disease may need to reduce your intake of foods like tomatoes, bananas, and oranges that are high in potassium. An expert in

nutrition can advise on proper portion amounts
and substitutes.

Seniors with Kidney disease can assist preserve good
kidney function and general health by planning meals and
controlling portions.

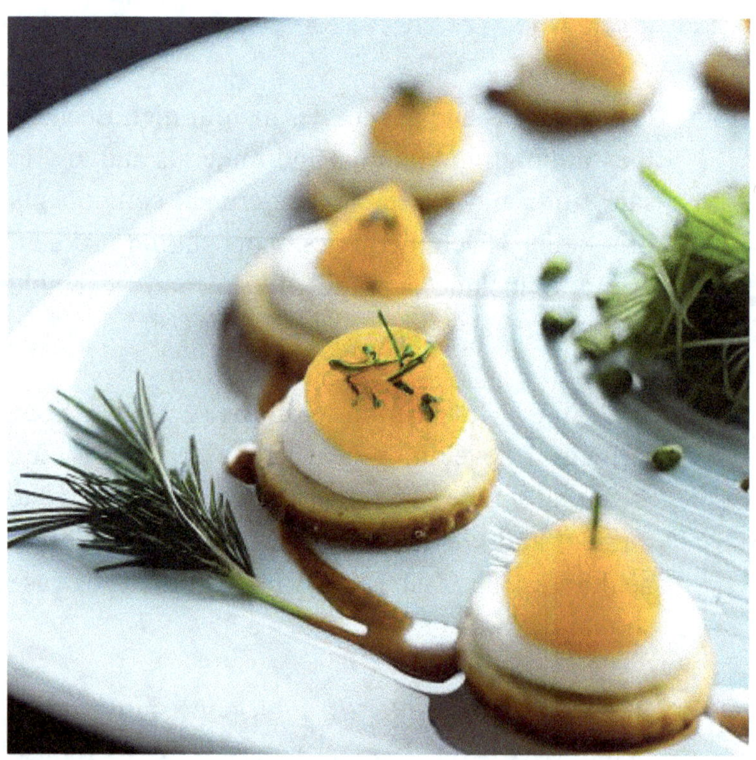

CHAPTER 2

BREAKFAST RECIPES:

Scrambled Eggs with Low-Sodium Ham and Spinach

Ingredients:

- 2 large eggs

- 1/4 cup low-sodium diced ham

- 1 cup fresh spinach leaves

- 1 tablespoon unsalted butter

- Salt and pepper to taste

Instruction

1. Crack the eggs into a small bowl and whisk with a fork until they're well-beaten.

2. Heat a non-stick skillet over medium heat and melt the butter.

3. Add the diced ham to the skillet and sauté for about a minute or until it's lightly browned.

4. Add the fresh spinach leaves to the skillet and sauté until wilted, about 2-3 minutes.

5. Pour the beaten eggs into the skillet and use a spatula to gently scramble them with the ham and spinach.

6. Continue to stir and cook the eggs until they're fully cooked and no longer runny, about 2-3 minutes.

7. Season with salt and pepper to taste.

8. Serve hot.

Oatmeal with Chopped Apples and Cinnamon

Ingredients:

- 1 cup old-fashioned rolled oats

- 2 cups water

- 1/4 teaspoon salt

- 1 medium apple, peeled and chopped

- 1/4 teaspoon ground cinnamon

- 1 tablespoon honey (optional)

Instructions

1. Combine the oats, water, and salt in a medium saucepan over medium-high heat.

2. Bring the mixture to a boil, then reduce the heat to medium-low and simmer for about 5-7 minutes or until the oats are tender and the mixture has thickened.

3. Stir in the chopped apple, ground cinnamon, and honey (if using).

4. Simmer for an additional 2-3 minutes or until the apple is softened and the oatmeal is heated through.

5. Remove from the heat and let the oatmeal cool for a few minutes before serving.

6. Serve hot, garnished with additional chopped apple and a sprinkle of cinnamon if desired.

Poached Eggs on Whole Grain Toast with Avocado

Ingredients:

- 2 slices of whole grain bread

- 2 eggs

- 1/2 avocado, sliced

- 1/4 teaspoon salt

- 1/4 teaspoon black pepper

- 1 teaspoon white vinegar

Instructions

1. Toast the whole grain bread to your liking.

2. While the bread is toasting, bring a medium pot of water to a simmer over medium heat.

3. Add the white vinegar to the water and stir.

4. Crack each egg into a small bowl.

5. Using a slotted spoon, create a whirlpool in the pot of simmering water.

6. Carefully slide each egg into the water and cook for 3-4 minutes, or until the whites are set but the yolks are still runny.

7. Using the slotted spoon, remove the eggs from the water and place them on a paper towel to drain off any excess water.

8. Place the sliced avocado on top of the toasted bread slices.

9. Gently place one poached egg on each slice of avocado toast.

10. Season with salt and pepper to taste.

11. Serve immediately.

Greek Yogurt with Berries and Walnuts

Ingredients:

- 1 cup plain Greek yogurt

- 1 cup mixed berries (such as blueberries, raspberries, and strawberries)

- 1/4 cup chopped walnuts

- 1 tablespoon honey

Instructions

1. In a small bowl, mix together the Greek yogurt and honey until well combined.

2. Place the mixed berries on top of the yogurt.

3. Sprinkle the chopped walnuts on top of the berries.

4. Serve immediately.

5. Optional: Drizzle additional honey on top for added sweetness.

Low-Sodium Vegetable Omelet with Whole Grain Toast

Ingredients:

- 2 large eggs
- 1/4 cup diced red bell pepper

- 1/4 cup diced green bell pepper

- 1/4 cup diced onion

- 1/4 cup sliced mushrooms

- 1 tablespoon unsalted butter

- Salt and pepper to taste

- 2 slices of whole grain toast

Instructions

1. Crack the eggs into a small bowl and whisk with a fork until they're well-beaten.

2. Heat a non-stick skillet over medium heat and melt the butter.

3. Add the diced bell peppers, onion, and mushrooms to the skillet and sauté for about 2-3 minutes or until they're slightly softened.

4. Pour the beaten eggs into the skillet and use a spatula to gently scramble them with the vegetables.

5. Continue to stir and cook the eggs until they're fully cooked and no longer runny, about 2-3 minutes.

6. Season with salt and pepper to taste.

7. Serve hot with two slices of whole grain toast on the side.

Recipe for Sweet Potato and Black Bean Breakfast Burrito

Ingredients:

- 1 medium sweet potato, peeled and diced

- 1/2 cup canned low-sodium black beans, drained and rinsed

- 1/4 cup diced red bell pepper

- 1/4 cup diced onion

- 1/4 teaspoon ground cumin

- 1/4 teaspoon chili powder

- Salt and pepper to taste

- 2 large eggs, scrambled

- 1/4 cup shredded low-fat cheddar cheese

- 2 large whole grain tortillas

Instructions

1. Preheat the oven to 400°F.

2. In a large bowl, toss the sweet potato, black beans, red bell pepper, onion, ground cumin, chili powder, salt, and pepper until well-combined.

3. Spread the sweet potato mixture in a single layer on a baking sheet and bake for 20-25 minutes or until the sweet potatoes are tender and lightly browned.

4. While the sweet potatoes are baking, scramble the eggs in a non-stick skillet until fully cooked and no longer runny.

5. Warm the tortillas in the microwave for 10-15 seconds.

6. Assemble the burritos by dividing the sweet potato mixture and scrambled eggs evenly between the two tortillas.

7. Sprinkle the shredded cheddar cheese on top of the sweet potato mixture and eggs.

8. Roll up the tortillas and serve immediately.

Low-Sodium Turkey Sausage and Vegetable Frittata

Ingredients:

- 8 large eggs

- 1/2 cup diced onion

- 1/2 cup diced red bell pepper

- 1/2 cup sliced mushrooms

- 4 ounces low-sodium turkey sausage, sliced

- 1/4 teaspoon salt

- 1/4 teaspoon black pepper

- 1 tablespoon unsalted butter

- 1/4 cup shredded low-fat cheddar cheese

Instructions

1. Preheat the oven to 350°F.

2. Crack the eggs into a large bowl and whisk with a fork until well-beaten.

3. Add the diced onion, red bell pepper, mushrooms, and sliced turkey sausage to the bowl and stir until everything is well-combined.

4. Season with salt and pepper to taste.

5. Melt the butter in an oven-safe non-stick skillet over medium heat.

6. Add the egg mixture to the skillet and cook for about 5-7 minutes or until the edges start to set.

7. Sprinkle the shredded cheddar cheese on top of the frittata.

8. Transfer the skillet to the preheated oven and bake for 10-12 minutes or until the eggs are fully set.

9. Remove from the oven and let the frittata cool for
    a few minutes before slicing and serving.

Homemade Granola with Low-Fat Milk or Yogurt

Ingredients:

- 2 cups old-fashioned rolled oats

- 1/2 cup chopped almonds

- 1/2 cup chopped walnuts

- 1/4 cup honey

- 1/4 cup unsalted butter, melted

- 1/2 teaspoon ground cinnamon

- 1/4 teaspoon salt

- 1/2 cup dried cranberries

- Low-fat milk or yogurt, for serving

Directions:

1. Preheat the oven to 350°F.

2. In a large bowl, mix together the oats, almonds, and walnuts.

3. In a separate small bowl, whisk together the honey, melted butter, cinnamon, and salt.

4. Pour the honey mixture over the oat mixture and stir until everything is well-coated.

5. Spread the mixture in a single layer on a baking sheet lined with parchment paper.

6. Bake for 20-25 minutes or until the granola is golden brown and fragrant.

7. Remove the baking sheet from the oven and let the granola cool completely.

8. Stir in the dried cranberries.

9. Serve the granola with low-fat milk or yogurt.

Cottage Cheese with Sliced Peaches and Almonds

Ingredients:

- 1 cup cottage cheese

- 1 ripe peach, sliced

- 1/4 cup sliced almonds

- 1 teaspoon honey (optional)

Instructions

1. Spoon the cottage cheese into a bowl.

2. Add the sliced peach on top of the cottage cheese.

3. Sprinkle the sliced almonds over the peach.

4. Drizzle honey over the top, if desired.

5. Serve and enjoy!

Low-Sodium Smoked Salmon on a Whole Grain Bagel with Cream Cheese

Ingredients:

- 1 whole grain bagel, sliced in half

- 2 ounces low-sodium smoked salmon

- 1 tablespoon light cream cheese

- 1 tablespoon chopped fresh chives

Instructions

1. Toast the bagel halves until lightly browned.

2. Spread the light cream cheese on both halves of the bagel.

3. Place the smoked salmon on top of the cream cheese on one half of the bagel.

4. Sprinkle the chopped fresh chives over the smoked salmon.

5. Top with the other half of the bagel.

6. Serve and enjoy!

Cheese and Capers Appetizer

Ingredients:

- 4 ounces cream cheese, softened

- 2 tablespoons capers, drained and chopped

- 1 tablespoon chopped fresh parsley

- 1/4 teaspoon black pepper

Instructions

1. In a small bowl, mix together the cream cheese, chopped capers, chopped fresh parsley, and black pepper until well-combined.

2. Transfer the mixture to a serving dish.

3. Serve with crackers or sliced vegetables as a dip or spread.

4. Enjoy!

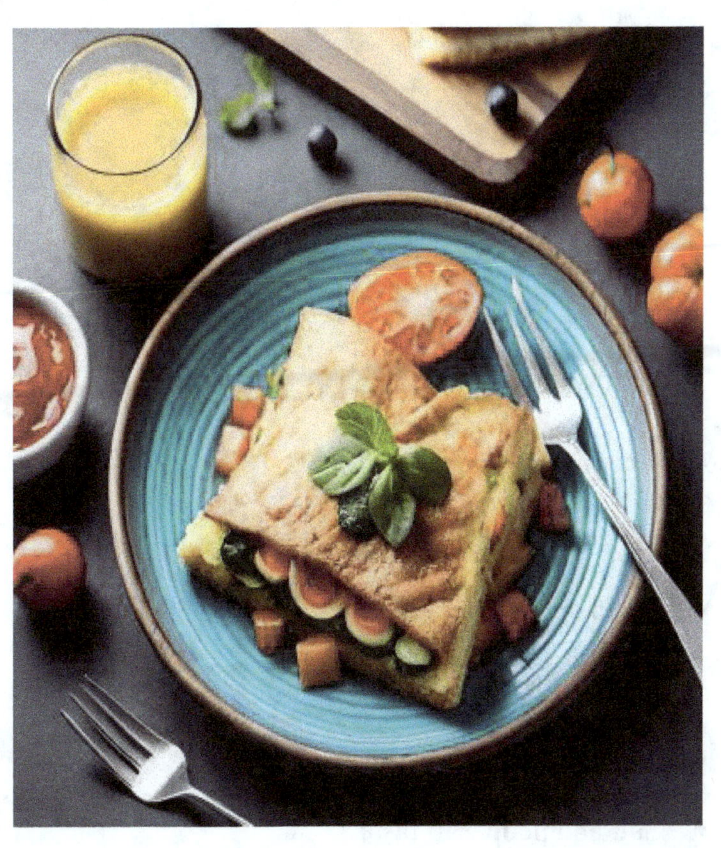

CHAPTER 3

LAUNCH RECIPES:

Grilled Chicken Salad

Ingredients:

- 2 boneless, skinless chicken breasts

- 4 cups mixed greens

- 1/2 cucumber, sliced

- 1 cup cherry tomatoes, halved

- 2 tablespoons olive oil

- 1 tablespoon apple cider vinegar

- Salt and pepper to taste

Instructions:

1. Preheat a grill or grill pan to medium-high heat.

2. Season the chicken breasts with salt and pepper.

3. Grill the chicken breasts for 6-7 minutes per side, or until the internal temperature reaches 165°F.

4. Remove the chicken from the grill and let it rest for 5 minutes.

5. In a small bowl, whisk together the olive oil and apple cider vinegar to make the dressing.

6. In a large bowl, toss the mixed greens, sliced cucumber, and halved cherry tomatoes with the dressing.

7. Slice the grilled chicken and arrange it on top of the salad.

8. Serve and enjoy!

Tuna Salad Lettuce Wraps

Ingredients:

- 2 cans of tuna, drained

- 1/4 cup celery, diced

- 1/4 cup red onion, diced

- 2 tablespoons light mayonnaise

- Salt and pepper to taste

- Lettuce leaves for wrapping

Instructions:

1. In a medium bowl, combine the drained tuna, diced celery, diced red onion, and light mayonnaise.

2. Season with salt and pepper to taste.

3. Mix well to combine all ingredients.

4. Take a lettuce leaf and spoon some of the tuna salad mixture into it.

5. Wrap the lettuce leaf around the mixture.

6. Repeat with remaining lettuce leaves and tuna salad mixture.

7. Serve and enjoy!

Black Bean Burger

Ingredients:

- 2 cans black beans, drained and rinsed

- 1/2 onion, diced

- 1/2 cup rolled oats

- 1/4 cup chopped fresh cilantro

- 1 tablespoon chili powder

- 1 teaspoon ground cumin

- 1/2 teaspoon salt

- 1/4 teaspoon black pepper

- 4 whole wheat buns

- Lettuce, tomato, and onion for topping

Instructions:

1. In a large bowl, mash the black beans with a fork or potato masher.

2. Add the diced onion, rolled oats, cilantro, chili powder, cumin, salt, and black pepper. Mix well to combine.

3. Form the mixture into 4 equal patties.

4. Heat a non-stick skillet over medium-high heat.

5. Cook the patties for 3-4 minutes per side, or until they are crispy and golden brown.

6. Serve each patty on a whole wheat bun with lettuce, tomato, and onion.

7. Enjoy!

Mediterranean Wrap

Ingredients:

- 1 whole wheat wrap

- 2 tablespoons hummus

- 1/4 cup roasted red peppers, sliced

- 1/4 cup artichoke hearts, chopped

- 1/4 cup crumbled feta cheese

- 2 ounces sliced chicken breast

Instructions:

1. Lay the whole wheat wrap flat on a plate.

2. Spread the hummus evenly on the wrap.

3. Arrange the roasted red peppers, artichoke hearts, and feta cheese on top of the hummus.

4. Add the sliced chicken breast on top.

5. Fold the bottom of the wrap up over the ingredients, then fold in the sides and roll tightly.

6. Cut the wrap in half and serve.

7. Enjoy!

Vegetable Frittata

Ingredients:

- 6 eggs

- 1/2 cup milk

- 1/2 teaspoon salt

- 1/4 teaspoon black pepper

- 1 tablespoon olive oil

- 1/2 zucchini, sliced

- 1/2 red bell pepper, diced

- 1/2 onion, diced

- 1/4 cup shredded cheese (optional)

- Salad greens for serving

Instructions:

1. Preheat the oven to 375°F.

2. In a medium bowl, whisk together the eggs, milk, salt, and black pepper.

3. Heat the olive oil in an oven-safe skillet over medium heat.

4. Add the zucchini, red bell pepper, and onion. Cook for 5-7 minutes, or until the vegetables are tender.

5. Pour the egg mixture into the skillet, covering the vegetables evenly.

6. Sprinkle the shredded cheese on top (if using).

7. Bake the frittata in the oven for 10-12 minutes, or until the eggs are set and the cheese is melted.

8. Serve the frittata with a side salad of mixed greens.

9. Enjoy!

Ingredients:

- 1 cup cooked quinoa

- 1/2 cucumber, diced

- 1 cup cherry tomatoes, halved

- 1/4 red onion, diced

- 1/4 cup chopped fresh parsley

- 2 tablespoons olive oil

- 1 tablespoon lemon juice

- Salt and pepper to taste

Instructions:

1. In a large bowl, combine the cooked quinoa, diced cucumber, halved cherry tomatoes, diced red onion, and chopped parsley.

2. In a small bowl, whisk together the olive oil and lemon juice to make the dressing.

3. Pour the dressing over the quinoa salad and toss to coat evenly.

4. Season with salt and pepper to taste.

5. Serve the quinoa salad at room temperature or chilled.

6. Enjoy!

Broiled Salmon

Ingredients:

- 4 salmon fillets (6 oz. each)

- 2 cloves garlic, minced

- 1 tablespoon chopped fresh dill

- Salt and pepper to taste

- 1 pound asparagus, trimmed

- 2 tablespoons olive oil

- 2 cups cooked brown rice

Instructions:

1. Preheat the broiler to high.

2. Line a baking sheet with aluminum foil and lightly coat with cooking spray.

3. Place the salmon fillets on the baking sheet and season with minced garlic, chopped dill, salt, and pepper.

4. Broil the salmon for 8-10 minutes, or until cooked through and flaky.

5. While the salmon is cooking, toss the trimmed asparagus with olive oil, salt, and pepper.

6. Roast the asparagus in the oven for 10-12 minutes, or until tender.

7. Serve each salmon fillet with a side of roasted asparagus and 1/2 cup of cooked brown rice.

8. Enjoy!

Shrimp Stir Fry

Ingredients:

- 1 pound shrimp, peeled and deveined

- 1 tablespoon cornstarch

- 1 tablespoon soy sauce

- 1/2 teaspoon garlic powder

- 1/2 teaspoon ground ginger

- 1/4 teaspoon black pepper

- 2 tablespoons vegetable oil

- 2 cups mixed vegetables (broccoli, bell peppers, snap peas)

- 2 cups cooked brown rice

Instructions:

1. In a medium bowl, combine the shrimp, cornstarch, soy sauce, garlic powder, ground ginger, and black pepper. Toss to coat the shrimp evenly.

2. Heat the vegetable oil in a large skillet or wok over high heat.

3. Add the mixed vegetables and stir-fry for 2-3 minutes, or until they are crisp-tender.

4. Add the shrimp to the skillet and stir-fry for an additional 2-3 minutes, or until the shrimp are cooked through.

5. Serve the shrimp stir fry over 1/2 cup of cooked brown rice.

6. Enjoy!

Chicken Vegetable Soup

Ingredients:

- 8 cups chicken broth

- 2 carrots, diced

- 2 celery stalks, diced

- 1 pound chicken breast, diced

- 2 cloves garlic, minced

- 1 teaspoon dried thyme

- 2 bay leaves

- Salt and pepper to taste

Instructions:

1. In a large pot, bring the chicken broth to a boil over high heat.

2. Add the diced carrots, celery, chicken breast, minced garlic, dried thyme, bay leaves, salt, and pepper to the pot.

3. Reduce the heat to low and let the soup simmer for 20-25 minutes, or until the vegetables are tender and the chicken is cooked through.

4. Remove the bay leaves and discard.

5. Serve the chicken vegetable soup hot and enjoy!

Turkey and Avocado Wrap

Ingredients:

- 1 whole wheat wrap

- 4 slices turkey breast

- 1/2 avocado, sliced

- 1 cup baby spinach

- 1 tablespoon Greek yogurt

- 1 teaspoon Dijon mustard

Instructions:

1. In a small bowl, mix together the Greek yogurt and Dijon mustard to make the dressing.

2. Lay the whole wheat wrap on a flat surface.

3. Layer the turkey breast, sliced avocado, and baby spinach on top of the wrap.

4. Drizzle the dressing over the ingredients.

5. Roll the wrap tightly and cut in half.
6. Serve the turkey and avocado wrap and enjoy!

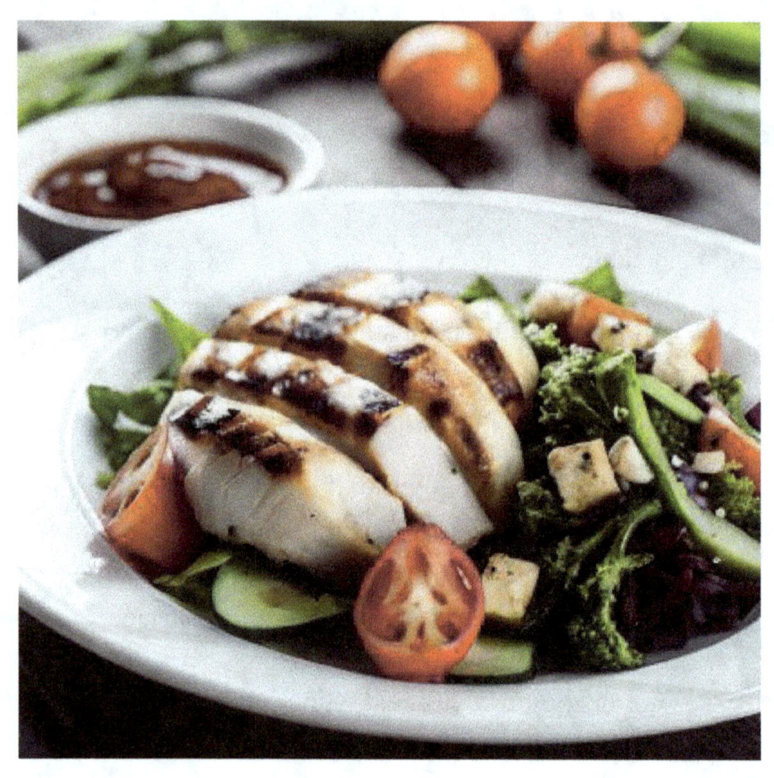

CHAPTER 4

DINNER RECIPES:

Baked Salmon with Roasted Vegetables

Ingredients:

- 4 salmon fillets

- 1 lemon, sliced

- 1 tablespoon fresh parsley, chopped

- 1 tablespoon fresh dill, chopped

- Salt and pepper, to taste

- 1 bunch asparagus, trimmed

- 1 red bell pepper, sliced

- 8 oz mushrooms, sliced

- 2 tablespoons olive oil

Instructions:

1. Preheat oven to 400°F (200°C).

2. Season salmon fillets with salt, pepper, and herbs. Place them on a baking sheet lined with parchment paper.

3. Arrange vegetables around the salmon and drizzle with olive oil. Season with salt and pepper.

4. Bake in the preheated oven for 15-20 minutes or until the salmon is cooked through and the vegetables are tender.

5. Serve hot.

Slow Cooker Beef Stew

Ingredients:

- 2 lbs lean beef stew meat, cut into cubes
- 3 carrots, chopped
- 3 celery stalks, chopped
- 2 potatoes, peeled and chopped
- 1 onion, chopped
- 4 garlic cloves, minced
- 2 cups low-sodium beef broth

- 1 tablespoon tomato paste

- 1 tablespoon Worcestershire sauce

- 1 teaspoon dried thyme

- 1 teaspoon dried rosemary

- Salt and pepper, to taste

- 2 tablespoons cornstarch

- 2 tablespoons cold water

Instructions:

1. In a slow cooker, combine the beef, vegetables, garlic, beef broth, tomato paste, Worcestershire sauce, and herbs. Season with salt and pepper.

2. Cook on low for 6-8 hours or until the beef is tender.

3. In a small bowl, whisk together cornstarch and cold water. Stir the mixture into the stew until thickened.

4. Serve hot with crusty bread or over cooked brown rice.

Grilled Chicken Skewers

Ingredients:

- 2 lbs boneless, skinless chicken breasts, cut into cubes

- 1/4 cup olive oil

- 3 garlic cloves, minced

- 2 tablespoons fresh lemon juice

- Salt and pepper, to taste

- 2 red bell peppers, cut into cubes

- 1 large red onion, cut into cubes

Instructions:

1. In a large bowl, whisk together olive oil, garlic, lemon juice, salt, and pepper.

2. Add chicken cubes to the marinade and toss to coat. Cover and refrigerate for at least 1 hour.
3. Preheat grill to medium-high heat. Thread chicken, bell peppers, and onion onto skewers.

4. Grill skewers for 10-12 minutes, turning occasionally, until the chicken is cooked through and the vegetables are charred and tender.

5. Serve hot with a side salad or grilled vegetables.

Ratatouille

Ingredients:

- 1 large eggplant, diced

- 2 zucchini, diced

- 2 bell peppers, diced

- 4 tomatoes, diced

- 1 onion, chopped

- 4 garlic cloves, minced

- 2 tablespoons olive oil

- 2 tablespoons fresh basil, chopped

- 1 tablespoon fresh thyme leaves

- Salt and pepper, to taste

Instructions:

1. In a large pot, heat olive oil over medium-high heat. Add onion and garlic and cook until softened.

2. Add eggplant, zucchini, and bell peppers to the pot. Season with salt and pepper and cook until vegetables are tender, about 10 minutes.

3. Add tomatoes, basil, and thyme to the pot. Cook for another 10 minutes, stirring occasionally.

4. Taste and adjust seasoning as needed. Serve hot as a side dish or over cooked quinoa or brown rice.

Lentil Soup

Ingredients:

- 1 onion, chopped

- 2 garlic cloves, minced

- 2 carrots, peeled and chopped

- 2 celery stalks, chopped

- 1 cup dried lentils, rinsed and drained

- 4 cups low-sodium vegetable broth

- 1 teaspoon ground cumin

- 1 teaspoon dried thyme

- Salt and pepper, to taste

Instructions:

1. In a large pot, heat olive oil over medium-high heat. Add onion and garlic and cook until softened.

2. Add carrots and celery to the pot and cook for another 5 minutes, stirring occasionally.

3. Add lentils, vegetable broth, cumin, thyme, salt, and pepper to the pot. Bring to a boil.

4. Reduce heat to low and simmer for 30-40 minutes, or until lentils are tender.

5. Taste and adjust seasoning as needed. Serve hot with a slice of whole-grain bread.

Pork Tenderloin with Roasted Sweet Potatoes

Ingredients:

- 1 lb pork tenderloin

- 2 tablespoons olive oil

- 1 tablespoon dried thyme

- 1 tablespoon dried rosemary

- Salt and pepper, to taste

- 2 large sweet potatoes, peeled and cubed

- 2 tablespoons honey

- 1 teaspoon ground cinnamon

- 1/2 teaspoon ground nutmeg

Instructions:

1. Preheat oven to 400°F (200°C). Line a baking sheet with parchment paper.

2. In a small bowl, mix together olive oil, thyme, rosemary, salt, and pepper. Rub the mixture over the pork tenderloin.

3. Place the pork tenderloin on the prepared baking sheet. Surround it with the cubed sweet potatoes.

4. In a small bowl, mix together honey, cinnamon, and nutmeg. Drizzle the mixture over the sweet potatoes.

5. Roast the pork tenderloin and sweet potatoes for 25-30 minutes, or until the pork is cooked through and the sweet potatoes are tender and caramelized.

6. Let the pork rest for a few minutes before slicing it. Serve hot with the roasted sweet potatoes.

Beef and Broccoli Stir Fry

Ingredients:

- 1 lb lean beef, thinly sliced

- 2 cups broccoli florets

- 1 onion, sliced

- 2 cloves garlic, minced

- 2 tbsp low-sodium soy sauce

- 1 tbsp olive oil

- Brown rice, cooked, for serving

Instructions:

1. Heat a large skillet or wok over high heat.

2. Add the olive oil and swirl to coat the bottom of the pan.

3. Add the beef and stir fry until browned on all sides, about 3-4 minutes.

4. Add the onion and garlic and continue to stir fry for another 2-3 minutes.

5. Add the broccoli and soy sauce to the pan, and stir fry for another 3-4 minutes until the broccoli is tender-crisp.

6. Serve the beef and broccoli over brown rice.

Grilled Eggplant and Zucchini Lasagna

Ingredients:

- 1 large eggplant, sliced into 1/4 inch rounds

- 2 medium zucchini, sliced into 1/4 inch rounds

- 2 cups low-sodium tomato sauce

- 1 cup low-fat ricotta cheese

- 1/4 cup grated Parmesan cheese

- 1/4 cup chopped fresh basil

- 1 tbsp olive oil

Instructions:

1. Preheat the grill to medium-high heat.

2. Brush the eggplant and zucchini slices with olive oil.

3. Grill the vegetables for 2-3 minutes per side, until lightly charred and tender.

4. In a 9x13 inch baking dish, spread a layer of tomato sauce on the bottom.

5. Add a layer of grilled eggplant slices, then a layer of grilled zucchini slices.

6. Top the vegetables with a layer of ricotta cheese, then another layer of tomato sauce.

7. Repeat the layers until all ingredients are used up, ending with a layer of tomato sauce.

8. Sprinkle Parmesan cheese over the top of the lasagna.

9. Bake in the oven at 375°F for 25-30 minutes, until bubbly and golden.

10. Garnish with chopped fresh basil before serving.

Lemon herb roasted chicken recipe

Ingredients:

- 4 bone-in, skin-on chicken breasts

- 2 tbsp olive oil

- 1 lemon, zested and juiced

- 2 cloves garlic, minced

- 1 tbsp chopped fresh rosemary

- 1 tbsp chopped fresh thyme

- Salt and pepper, to taste

- 4 carrots, peeled and cut into large pieces

- 4 potatoes, peeled and cut into large pieces

Instructions:

1. Preheat the oven to 375°F (190°C).

2. In a small bowl, whisk together the olive oil, lemon zest and juice, garlic, rosemary, thyme, salt, and pepper.

3. Place the chicken breasts in a baking dish and brush with the lemon herb mixture, making sure to coat both sides.

4. Add the carrots and potatoes to the dish, and toss with any remaining lemon herb mixture.

5. Roast in the oven for 45-50 minutes, or until the chicken is cooked through and the vegetables are tender.

6. Serve hot and enjoy!

Turkey chili recipe

Ingredients:

- 1 pound ground turkey

- 1 onion, diced

- 2 cloves garlic, minced

- 1 bell pepper, diced

- 1 can kidney beans, drained and rinsed

- 1 can diced tomatoes

- 2 tbsp chili powder

- 1 tsp cumin

- Salt and pepper, to taste

- Brown rice, for serving

Instructions

1. Heat a large pot over medium-high heat. Add the ground turkey and cook until browned, breaking it up with a wooden spoon as it cooks.

2. Add the onion, garlic, and bell pepper to the pot and cook until the vegetables are softened, about 5 minutes.

3. Add the kidney beans, diced tomatoes, chili powder, cumin, salt, and pepper to the pot, and stir to combine.

4. Bring the chili to a boil, then reduce the heat to low and let it simmer for 20-30 minutes, until the flavors have melded together and the chili has thickened slightly.

5. Serve the chili hot, over a bed of brown rice, and enjoy!

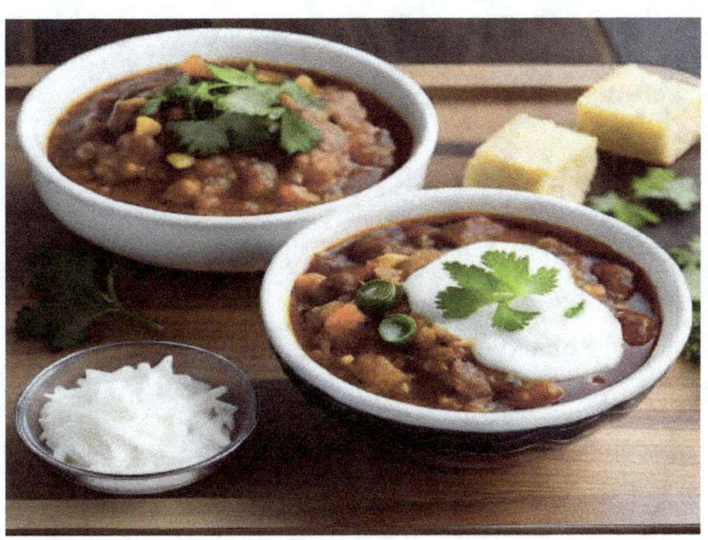

CHAPTER 5

SNACKS AND DESSERT RECIPES:

Roasted Chickpeas

Ingredients:

- 1 can of chickpeas, drained and rinsed

- 1 tablespoon of olive oil

- 1/4 teaspoon of salt

- 1/4 teaspoon of garlic powder

Instructions:

1. Preheat oven to 400°F.

2. Pat chickpeas dry with a paper towel.

3. Toss chickpeas with olive oil, salt, and garlic powder.

4. Spread chickpeas in a single layer on a baking sheet.

5. Bake for 20-30 minutes, or until crispy.

Ingredients:

- 1 medium sweet potato, peeled and sliced thinly

- 1 tablespoon of olive oil

- 1/4 teaspoon of salt

Instructions:

- Preheat oven to 375°F.

- Toss sweet potato slices with olive oil and salt.

- Place sweet potato slices in a single layer on a baking sheet.

- Bake for 20-30 minutes, or until crispy.

Ingredients:

- 1 cup of sliced strawberries

- 1 cup of diced pineapple

- 1 cup of sliced bananas

- 1 cup of blueberries

- 1/4 cup of honey

- 1 tablespoon of lime juice

Instructions:

1. Combine strawberries, pineapple, bananas, and blueberries in a large bowl.

2. In a separate bowl, whisk together honey and lime juice.

3. Pour honey-lime dressing over fruit and toss to coat.

Rice Pudding

Ingredients:

- 2 cups of cooked white rice

- 2 cups of unsweetened almond milk

- 1/4 cup of honey

- 1 teaspoon of vanilla extract

- 1/2 teaspoon of ground cinnamon

Instructions:

1. In a large saucepan, combine cooked rice, almond milk, honey, vanilla extract, and cinnamon.

2. Bring mixture to a boil over medium heat, stirring occasionally.

3. Reduce heat to low and simmer for 20-25 minutes, or until mixture thickens.

4. Serve warm or chilled.

Apple Chips

Ingredients:

- 2 apples, cored and thinly sliced

- 1/2 teaspoon of ground cinnamon

Instructions:

1. Preheat oven to 225°F.

2. Toss apple slices with cinnamon.

3. Place apple slices in a single layer on a baking sheet.

4. Bake for 2-3 hours, or until crispy.

Greek Yogurt with Berries

Ingredients:

- 1 cup of plain Greek yogurt

- 1/2 cup of sliced strawberries

- 1/2 cup of blueberries

- 1 tablespoon of honey

Instructions:

1. In a bowl, combine Greek yogurt, strawberries, blueberries, and honey.

2. Mix well and serve.

Chocolate Chia Pudding

Ingredients:

1/4 cup of chia seeds

1 cup of unsweetened almond milk

1 tablespoon of cocoa powder

1 tablespoon of honey

1/2 teaspoon of vanilla extract

Instructions:

1. In a large bowl, combine chia seeds, almond milk, cocoa powder, honey, and vanilla extract.

2. Stir well and let sit in the refrigerator for at least 30 minutes, or until pudding thickens.

3. Serve chilled.

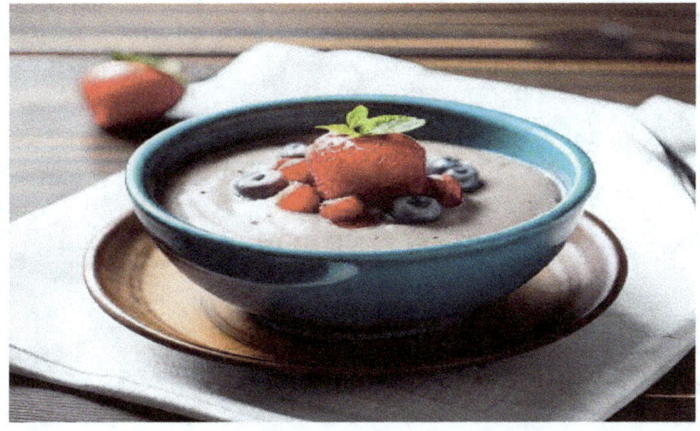

CHAPTER 6

SOUPS AND STEW:

Low-sodium vegetable soup recipe

Ingredients:

- 1 tablespoon olive oil

- 1 onion, chopped

- 2 garlic cloves, minced

- 2 carrots, chopped

- 2 celery stalks, chopped

- 1 zucchini, chopped

- 1 red bell pepper, chopped

- 4 cups low-sodium vegetable broth

- 1 can (14.5 ounces) diced tomatoes, undrained

- 1 teaspoon dried thyme

- Salt and pepper, to taste

- 2 cups chopped fresh spinach

Instructions

1. Heat the olive oil in a large pot over medium heat. Add the onion and garlic and cook until soft and fragrant.

2. Add the carrots, celery, zucchini, and red bell pepper and cook for another 5 minutes, stirring occasionally.

3. Add the vegetable broth, diced tomatoes, thyme, salt, and pepper. Bring to a boil, then reduce heat and simmer for 15-20 minutes, or until the vegetables are tender.

4. Stir in the chopped spinach and cook for another 5 minutes, or until the spinach is wilted.

5. Serve hot and enjoy.

Creamy asparagus soup recipe

Ingredients:

- 2 tablespoons unsalted butter

- 1 onion, chopped

- 2 garlic cloves, minced

- 1 pound asparagus, trimmed and cut into 1-inch pieces

- 4 cups low-sodium chicken or vegetable broth

- 1 cup low-fat milk

- 1/4 cup heavy cream

- Salt and pepper, to taste

- Chopped fresh chives or parsley, for garnish (optional)

Instructions

1. Melt the butter in a large pot over medium heat. Add the onion and garlic and cook until soft and fragrant.

2. Add the asparagus and cook for another 5 minutes, stirring occasionally.

3. Add the broth and bring to a boil, then reduce heat and simmer for 15-20 minutes, or until the asparagus is tender.

4. Puree the soup in batches in a blender or food processor until smooth.

5. Return the soup to the pot and stir in the milk and cream. Heat over medium heat until heated through, but do not boil.

6. Season with salt and pepper, to taste.

7. Serve hot, garnished with chopped fresh chives or parsley, if desired.

Chicken and vegetable soup recipe

Ingredients:

- 1 tablespoon olive oil

- 1 onion, chopped

- 2 garlic cloves, minced

- 2 carrots, chopped

- 2 celery stalks, chopped

- 6 cups low-sodium chicken broth

- 1 pound boneless, skinless chicken breast, cut into bite-size pieces

- 1 zucchini, chopped

- 1 can (14.5 ounces) diced tomatoes, undrained

- 1 teaspoon dried thyme

- Salt and pepper, to taste

- 2 cups chopped fresh spinach

Instructions

1. Heat the olive oil in a large pot over medium heat. Add the onion and garlic and cook until soft and fragrant.

2. Add the carrots, celery, and chicken and cook for another 5 minutes, stirring occasionally.

3. Add the chicken broth, zucchini, diced tomatoes, thyme, salt, and pepper. Bring to a boil, then reduce heat and simmer for 15-20 minutes, or until the vegetables are tender and the chicken is cooked through.

4. Stir in the chopped spinach and cook for another
    5 minutes, or until the spinach is wilted.

5. Serve hot and enjoy.

Ingredients:

- 2 tablespoons unsalted butter

- 1 onion, chopped

- 2 garlic cloves, minced

- 2 cans (14.5 ounces each) low-sodium diced
  tomatoes, undrained

- 4 cups low-sodium chicken or vegetable broth

- 1/4 cup heavy cream

- Salt and pepper, to taste

- Chopped fresh basil or parsley, for garnish
  (optional)

Instructions

1. Melt the butter in a large pot over medium heat. Add the onion and garlic and cook until soft and fragrant.

2. Add the diced tomatoes and broth and bring to a boil, then reduce heat and simmer for 15-20 minutes.

3. Puree the soup in batches in a blender or food processor until smooth.

4. Return the soup to the pot and stir in the heavy cream. Heat over medium heat until heated through, but do not boil.

5. Season with salt and pepper, to taste.

6. Serve hot, garnished with chopped fresh basil or parsley, if desired.

Minestrone soup recipe

Ingredients:

- 1 tablespoon olive oil

- 1 onion, chopped

- 2 garlic cloves, minced

- 2 carrots, chopped

- 2 celery stalks, chopped

- 1 zucchini, chopped

- 1 can (14.5 ounces) diced tomatoes, undrained

- 4 cups low-sodium vegetable broth

- 1 can (15 ounces) low-sodium kidney beans, drained and rinsed

- 1 teaspoon dried basil

- Salt and pepper, to taste

- 1/2 cup dry elbow pasta

- 2 cups chopped fresh spinach

Instructions

1. Heat the olive oil in a large pot over medium heat. Add the onion and garlic and cook until soft and fragrant.

2. Add the carrots, celery, zucchini, and diced
    tomatoes and cook for another 5 minutes, stirring
    occasionally.

3. Add the vegetable broth, kidney beans, basil, salt,
    and pepper. Bring to a boil, then reduce heat and
    simmer for 15-20 minutes, or until the vegetables
    are tender.

4. Stir in the elbow pasta and cook for another 10-
    12 minutes, or until the pasta is cooked al dente.

5. Stir in the chopped spinach and cook for another
    5 minutes, or until the spinach is wilted.

6. Serve hot and enjoy.

Beef and barley soup recipe

Ingredients:

- 1 tablespoon olive oil

- 1 onion, chopped

- 2 garlic cloves, minced

- 1 pound lean beef stew meat, cut into bite-size
  pieces

- 4 cups low-sodium beef broth

- 1/2 cup pearl barley

- 2 carrots, chopped

- 2 celery stalks, chopped

- 1 teaspoon dried thyme

- Salt and pepper, to taste

- Chopped fresh parsley, for garnish (optional)

Instructions

1. Heat the olive oil in a large pot over medium heat. Add the onion and garlic and cook until soft and fragrant.

2. Add the beef and cook for another 5-7 minutes, or until browned on all sides.

3. Add the beef broth, barley, carrots, celery, thyme, salt, and pepper. Bring to a boil, then reduce heat and simmer for 1-1 1/2 hours, or until the beef and barley are tender.

4. Serve hot, garnished with chopped fresh parsley, if desired.

Ingredients:

- 1 tablespoon olive oil

- 1 onion, chopped

- 2 garlic cloves, minced

- 2 carrots, chopped

- 2 celery stalks, chopped

- 1 cup dried brown lentils, rinsed and drained

- 4 cups low-sodium vegetable broth

- 1 can (14.5 ounces) diced tomatoes, undrained

- 1 teaspoon dried thyme

- Salt and pepper, to taste

- 2 cups chopped fresh spinach

Instructions

1. Heat the olive oil in a large pot over medium heat. Add the onion and garlic and cook until soft and fragrant.

2. Add the carrots, celery, and lentils and cook for another 5 minutes, stirring occasionally.

3. Add the vegetable broth, diced tomatoes, thyme, salt, and pepper. Bring to a boil, then reduce heat and simmer for 30-40 minutes, or until the lentils are tender.

4. Stir in the chopped spinach and cook for another 5 minutes, or until the spinach is wilted.

5. Serve hot and enjoy.

Creamy potato soup recipe

Ingredients:

- 4 large potatoes, peeled and cubed

- 1 onion, chopped

- 2 garlic cloves, minced

- 4 cups low-sodium vegetable broth

- 1 cup low-fat milk or cream

- 1 teaspoon dried thyme

- Salt and pepper, to taste

- Chopped fresh chives, for garnish (optional)

Instructions

1. In a large pot, combine the potatoes, onion, garlic, and vegetable broth. Bring to a boil, then reduce heat and simmer for 20-25 minutes, or until the potatoes are tender.

2. Remove the pot from the heat and let cool slightly. Use an immersion blender or transfer the soup to a blender and puree until smooth.

3. Return the soup to the pot and add the milk or cream, thyme, salt, and pepper. Heat over low heat, stirring occasionally, until heated through.

4. Serve hot, garnished with chopped fresh chives, if desired.

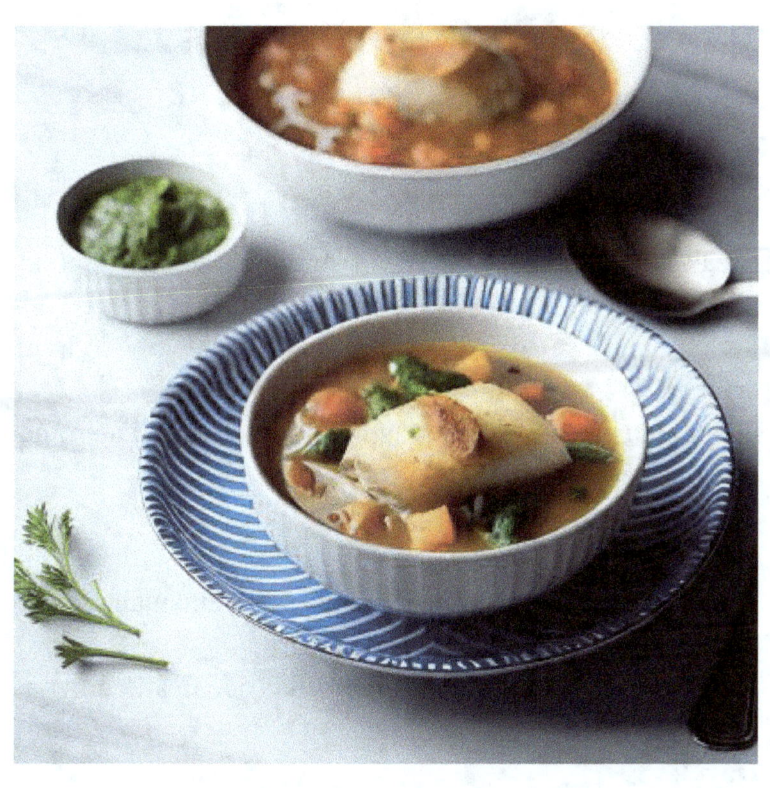

CHAPTER 7

21 DAYS MEAL PLAN:

Day 1:
Breakfast: Oatmeal with sliced strawberries and almond milk
Lunch: Tuna salad with mixed greens and low-sodium crackers
Dinner: Grilled chicken breast with roasted asparagus and brown rice

Day 2:
Breakfast: Greek yogurt with blueberries and walnuts
Lunch: Lentil soup with a side salad
Dinner: Baked salmon with steamed broccoli and quinoa

Day 3:
Breakfast: Scrambled eggs with spinach and whole wheat toast
Lunch: Chicken and vegetable stir-fry with brown rice
Dinner: Turkey chili with a side of low-sodium cornbread

Day 4:
Breakfast: Smoothie made with mixed berries, spinach, and almond milk
Lunch: Grilled chicken and vegetable kabobs with brown rice

Dinner: Baked sweet potato with black beans, salsa, and avocado

Day 5:
Breakfast: Low-sodium cottage cheese with peach slices and whole grain toast
Lunch: Vegetable and bean soup with a side salad
Dinner: Grilled shrimp with zucchini noodles and tomato sauce

Day 6:
Breakfast: Scrambled eggs with low-sodium ham and whole wheat toast
Lunch: Quinoa and black bean salad with mixed greens
Dinner: Baked chicken breast with roasted Brussels sprouts and sweet potato

Day 7:
Breakfast: Greek yogurt with mixed berries and almonds
Lunch: Turkey and vegetable wrap with low-sodium tortilla and side of fruit
Dinner: Grilled pork tenderloin with steamed green beans and brown rice

Day 8:
Breakfast: Smoothie made with banana, spinach, and almond milk

Lunch: Grilled chicken salad with mixed greens and low-sodium dressing

Dinner: Baked tilapia with roasted cauliflower and quinoa

Day 9:
Breakfast: Omelet with low-sodium cheese and vegetables
Lunch: Lentil and vegetable stew with a side of fruit
Dinner: Turkey meatballs with spaghetti squash and tomato sauce

Day 10:
Breakfast: Low-sodium cottage cheese with pineapple and whole grain toast
Lunch: Grilled shrimp salad with mixed greens and low-sodium dressing
Dinner: Baked chicken thighs with roasted carrots and brown rice

Day 11:
Breakfast: Smoothie made with mixed berries, spinach, and almond milk
Lunch: Chicken and vegetable stir-fry with brown rice
Dinner: Baked salmon with steamed broccoli and quinoa

Day 12:
Breakfast: Greek yogurt with blueberries and walnuts

Lunch: Tuna salad with mixed greens and low-sodium crackers

Dinner: Grilled chicken breast with roasted asparagus and brown rice

Day 13:

Breakfast: Scrambled eggs with spinach and whole wheat toast

Lunch: Lentil soup with a side salad

Dinner: Baked sweet potato with black beans, salsa, and avocado

Day 14:

Breakfast: Low-sodium cottage cheese with peach slices and whole grain toast

Lunch: Vegetable and bean soup with a side salad

Dinner: Grilled shrimp with zucchini noodles and tomato sauce

Day 15:

Breakfast: Smoothie made with banana, spinach, and almond milk

Lunch: Quinoa and black bean salad with mixed greens

Dinner: Baked chicken breast with roasted Brussels sprouts and sweet potato

Day 16:

Breakfast: Oatmeal with sliced strawberries and almond milk
Lunch: Turkey and vegetable wrap with low-sodium tortilla and side of fruit
Dinner: Grilled pork tenderlo

Day 17:
Breakfast: Greek yogurt with mixed berries and almonds
Lunch: Grilled chicken salad with mixed greens and low-sodium dressing
Dinner: Baked tilapia with roasted cauliflower and quinoa

Day 18:
Breakfast: Smoothie made with mixed berries, spinach, and almond milk
Lunch: Chicken and vegetable stir-fry with brown rice
Dinner: Baked salmon with steamed broccoli and quinoa

Day 19:
Breakfast: Scrambled eggs with low-sodium ham and whole wheat toast
Lunch: Lentil and vegetable stew with a side of fruit
Dinner: Turkey meatballs with spaghetti squash and tomato sauce

Day 20:
Breakfast: Low-sodium cottage cheese with pineapple and whole grain toast

Lunch: Grilled shrimp salad with mixed greens and low-sodium dressing
Dinner: Baked chicken thighs with roasted carrots and brown rice

Day 21:
Breakfast: Omelet with low-sodium cheese and vegetables
Lunch: Tuna salad with mixed greens and low-sodium crackers
Dinner: Grilled chicken breast with roasted asparagus and brown rice

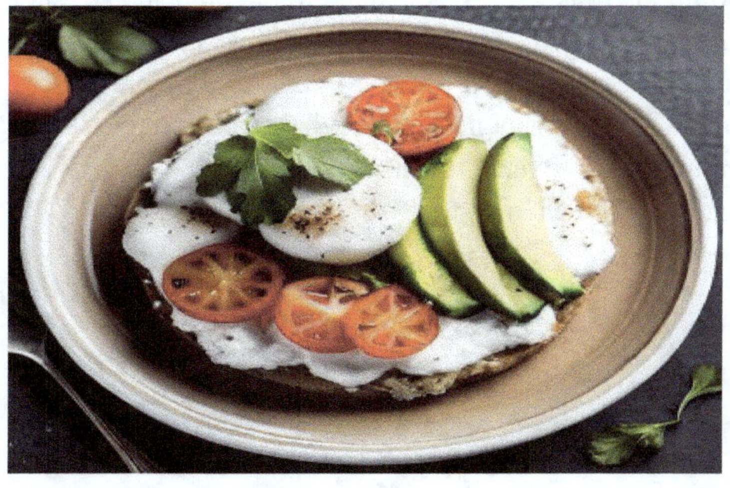

CONCLUSION

In conclusion, a kidney-friendly diet is an essential aspect of managing kidney disease, especially for seniors. By following a diet that is low in sodium, potassium, and phosphorus, seniors can help slow the progression of kidney disease and reduce the risk of complications. It is important for seniors to work closely with a registered dietitian to develop a personalized meal plan that meets their individual dietary needs and preferences.

In addition to following a kidney-friendly diet, seniors should also take steps to manage their fluid intake, stay physically active, and avoid smoking and excessive alcohol consumption. By taking a comprehensive approach to managing kidney disease, seniors can improve their overall health and well-being and live a longer, healthier life.

Final tips and advice for following a kidney diet as a senior.

1. Work with a registered dietitian: A registered dietitian can help you develop a personalized meal plan that meets your individual dietary needs and preferences. They can also provide guidance on portion sizes, label reading, and dining out.

2. Stay hydrated: While it's important to limit your fluid intake if you have kidney disease, it's still important to stay hydrated. Talk to your healthcare provider about how much fluid you should be drinking each day, and find creative ways to stay hydrated, such as eating water-rich fruits and vegetables.

3. Be mindful of protein intake: Protein is an important nutrient, but seniors with kidney disease may need to limit their protein intake. Talk to your dietitian about how much protein you should be eating each day, and choose high-quality sources of protein, such as lean meats, poultry, fish, and plant-based sources.

4. Limit processed and packaged foods: Many processed and packaged foods are high in sodium, phosphorus, and other nutrients that seniors with kidney disease should limit. Instead, focus on eating fresh, whole foods, such as fruits, vegetables, whole grains, and lean proteins.

5. Take medications as prescribed: Some medications can interact with certain foods or nutrients, so it's important to take your medications as prescribed and to talk to your

healthcare provider or pharmacist about any potential interactions.

6. Stay active: Regular physical activity can help improve kidney function, reduce the risk of chronic health conditions, and improve overall health and well-being. Talk to your healthcare provider about how much physical activity is safe for you, and find activities that you enjoy and can do safely.

Resources and support for living with kidney diseases

Although coping with renal disease can be difficult, there are numerous tools and sources of support that can be used to alleviate the burden on patients and their loved ones. Here are a few instances:

1. The National Kidney Foundation (NKF) is a nonprofit organization whose goal is to make kidney disease patients' lives better. They provide a range of resources, such as support services, advocacy, and education.

2.

3. The American Kidney Fund (AKF) helps people with Kidney disease who are having financial difficulties with their medical bills or other connected expenses.

4. Kidney Community Emergency Response (KCER) Program: In the case of an emergency or disaster, the KCER Program offers information and resources to people with kidney disease and their families.

5. The Renal Support Network (RSN) is a nonprofit group that offers assistance and information to people with kidney illness and their families.

6. Local support groups: Kidney disease sufferers and the people they love can find help in many local communities. These organizations can offer a sense of belonging and support, as well as practical tools and data.

7. Healthcare professionals: As you navigate living with kidney illness, your healthcare team can offer invaluable advice and support. They can assist you in managing your condition and, if necessary, put you in touch with the right resources and support.

Keep in mind that you are not experiencing renal illness alone. At any time you require it, ask for assistance and support.

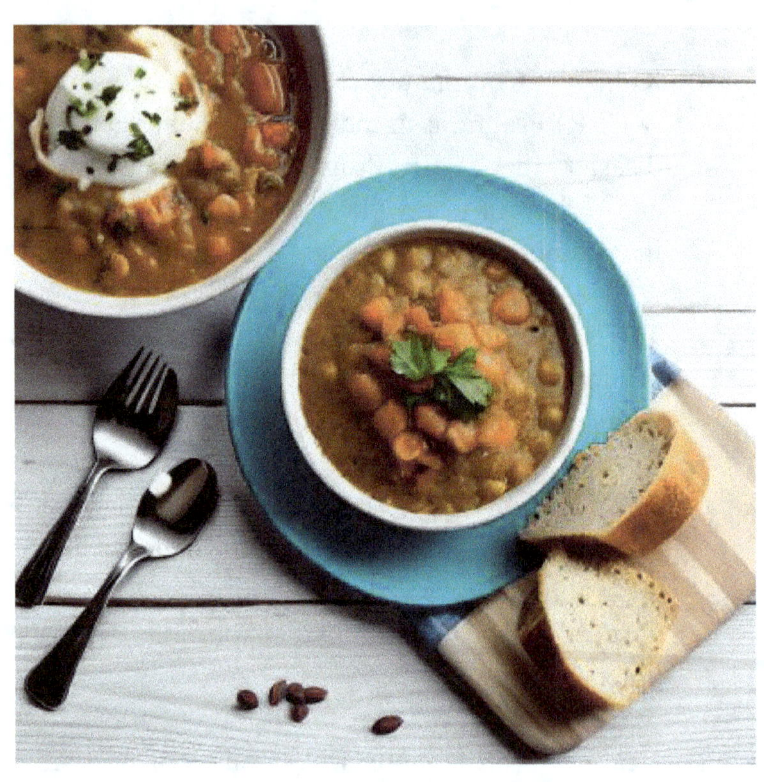

www.ingramcontent.com/pod-product-compliance
Lightning Source LLC
Chambersburg PA
CBHW051825250726
48659CB00005B/1681